all about **LOW-FODMAP DIET & IBS**

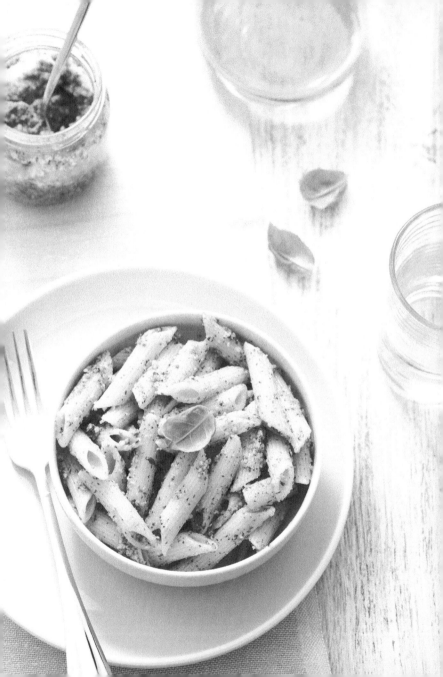

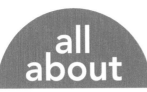

LOW-FODMAP DIET & IBS

A VERY QUICK GUIDE

LITTLE BOOKS ON **BIG** IDEAS

ISBN: Print 978-1-62315-538-4 | eBook 978-1-62315-539-1

Contents

LOW-FODMAP DIET RECIPES

The Low-FODMAP Diet

Trying the Low-FODMAP diet will provide you with valuable tools to make food choices that enhance your life and health.

If you, a loved one, or someone you care for are among the 25 to 45 million Americans suffering from irritable bowel syndrome (IBS), then your daily food choices probably cause more than physical symptoms. Flare-ups of the condition can trigger feelings of anxiety, embarrassment, and isolation, too. Even worse, finding adequate medical treatments is often challenging and expensive.

Fortunately, the low-FODMAP diet offers a way out of this suffering. This very quick guide contains all of the tools you need to regain some control over the condition and free yourself from the physical and emotional distress caused by IBS.

What's a FODMAP? FODMAP is an acronym for "fermentable oligosaccharides, disaccharides, monosaccharides, and polyols." In simple terms, a low-FODMAP diet restricts certain types of carbohydrates, providing symptomatic relief for many people with IBS. By minimizing your consumption of foods containing FODMAPs, you significantly reduce your chances of experiencing unpleasant symptoms like bloating, cramps, and diarrhea.

Combining a standard elimination diet strategy with FODMAP foods instead of allergens has become a successful strategy for managing IBS. If you suffer from IBS, trying the Low-FODMAP diet will provide you with valuable tools to make food choices that enhance your life and health, and could be the answer you seek for relief.

You might feel intimidated by a diet that restricts the foods you are allowed to eat. Many aspects of family, social, and cultural life center around food, and by limiting your diet, it may seem as though you are limiting your lifestyle. The good news is that eating a low-FODMAP diet doesn't mean consuming bland, mushy foods. To get you started, this book contains 21 delicious and enjoyable low-FODMAP recipes that appeal to the palate without disrupting the gut. In addition, it provides the following tools to help you achieve a low-FODMAP lifestyle that is both sustainable and enjoyable:

- Lists of high- and low-FODMAP ingredients that show what you can and cannot consume safely
- Detailed information about low-FODMAP diets to help you understand the hows and whys of the lifestyle
- A guide to help you identify trigger foods and track your symptoms
- Step-by-step recipes that make food preparation simple and easy

With so many tasty dishes to choose from, your daily food choices will soon be driven by delicious flavors, not problem reactions. Get ready to enjoy a satisfying and symptom-free lifestyle.

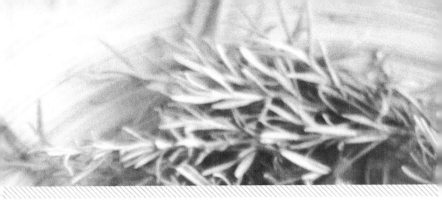

PART ONE

LOW-FODMAP
DIET BASICS

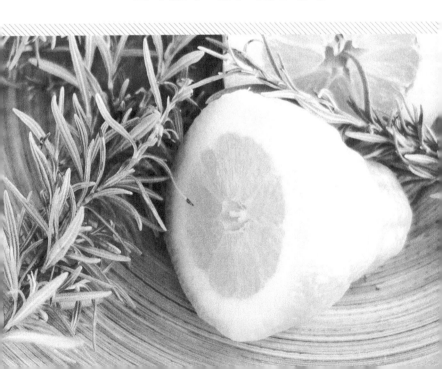

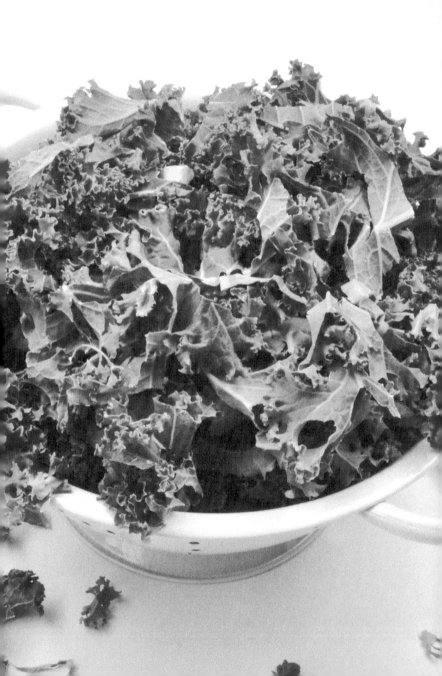

WHAT IS THE LOW-FODMAP DIET?

For many Americans, the word diet has negative connotations, drawing to mind a period of temporary deprivation and hard work in pursuit of weight loss. The low-FODMAP lifestyle isn't

your typical diet experience. It is a customizable eating plan created to allow IBS sufferers like you or your loved one to make positive dietary changes, ensuring a more healthy future.

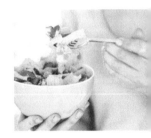

If you have IBS, then you already know the discomfort it can cause, with painful and embarrassing gastrointestinal symptoms, including gas, cramping, bloating, and diarrhea. You may also be suffering from a reduced quality of life, because making plans can be difficult when you never know whether you will experience symptoms that require you to stay close to home. The low-FODMAP diet offers you the ability to live your life as you did before you had IBS: free from gastrointestinal discomfort and embarrassment. It is a positive lifestyle change that allows you to reduce your symptoms and improve your quality of life.

The science behind FODMAPS

IBS is considered to be a functional bowel disorder which means there are no apparent anatomical, infectious, or metabolic issues, but symptoms still persist, negatively impacting the quality of life and health. Since there is no definitive cause for IBS, it is very difficult for health care providers to craft a treatment that will work effectively. The cause (or causes) of IBS is not fully understood, so most doctors simply address the symptoms with medication, digestive treatments such as laxatives or bulking agents, and advice on lifestyle choices.

In the 2000s, Peter R. Gibson and Susan J. Shepherd, two researchers at Monash University in Australia, set out to explore

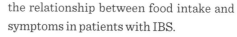

the relationship between food intake and symptoms in patients with IBS.

What they discovered was an approach to eating that offered significant symptomatic relief in 75 percent of the people in the study. By making the same strategic changes in your diet, you may be able to experience a similar reduction in or elimination of the discomfort associated with IBS.

When you see the list of foods that are considered high-FODMAPs, you might wonder what they have in common. There are both healthy foods and junk foods in both high- and low-FODMAP groups. The answer is that they all contain carbohydrates.

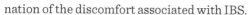

Carbohydrates—simple and complex carbs and fiber—are concentrated in plant foods. Simple carbohydrates are listed on packaged food nutrition labels as sugars, which can be the sugars naturally found in milk, fruits, and vegetables or processed and refined sugars and syrups. Complex carbohydrates found in grains and legumes as well as in fruits and vegetables are sometimes referred to as starch. These carbohydrates are broken down by bacteria in the gut into the nutrients our bodies need.

How FODMAPs Affect Digestion

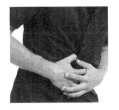

FODMAPs are a group of natural sugars (carbohydrates) that are poorly absorbed by the body. Not all carbohydrates are FOD-MAPs, so it is important to look closer at what sugars fall into this group.

Fructose (fermentable oligosaccharides): includes apples, pears, mango, watermelon, cherries, fruit juice, honey, agave, and high-fructose corn syrup

Oligosaccharides (GOS): includes non-canned lentils, non-canned garbanzo beans (chickpeas), hummus, kidney beans, pinto beans, peas, whole soybeans

Lactose (disaccharides): includes milk and milk products from cows, goats, and sheep

Fructans (monosaccharides): includes wheat, rye, graham flour, rye, onions, artichoke, Brussels sprouts, broccoli, cabbage, fennel, garlic, leeks, okra, red cabbage, radicchio, shallots, and watermelon

Polyols: includes glycerol, isomalt, maltitol, mannitol, sorbitol, xylitol, apples, apricots, cherries, peaches, nectarines, pears, plums, prunes, avocados, blackberries, lychees, cauliflower, and mushrooms

If FODMAPS make it into the large intestine they can cause bloating and gas when fermented by bacteria in the gut. Diarrhea can also develop due to an influx of fluid when there is excess sugar in the large intestine.

In addition, there are some carbohydrates that humans are not able to digest, known as fiber. Even though fiber doesn't supply nutrients to the body, it is still important to our health and digestive system. Soluble fibers have been shown to be part of keeping cholesterol levels and plaque low. Insoluble fiber has long been known for its ability to keep us regular.

All these different types of carbohydrates share a characteristic: Once they arrive in the gut, they begin to ferment. If something happens to disrupt the amount of bacteria at work in the gut or the amount of time a food spends in the gut, there can be several consequences.

Someone with a functional digestive disorder may be unable to digest certain carbohydrates for a variety of reasons. They may lack a specific enzyme or enough bacteria in the small intestine, for example. When carbohydrates aren't digested in the small intestine—a condition referred to as malabsorption—the bacteria in the large intestine suddenly find themselves with a bounty of the things they love to eat. The by-products of the bacterial feasting include acids, alcohols, and carbon dioxide, the same process that happens when yeast bread rises or beer is brewed. Since this is happening inside your gut, the gas is trapped. That's why some foods can make you not only feel but look bloated.

This is unpleasant enough, but it gets more complicated. Once fermentation is under way, it changes the pH of the gut, opening the door for a host of additional symptoms, ranging from gas and belching to inflammation and acid reflux. The rapid growth of the bacteria puts stress on the membranes lining the intestines and gut, and they become permeable. Important nutrients are able to leak out of the digestive tract before they are properly digested and absorbed.

In addition, these compounds are considered "osmotic" since they can attract and hold moisture. Bakers and pastry chefs take advantage of sugar's ability to attract and hold moisture to keep baked goods moist and flavorful for a long time. When someone sensitive to FODMAPs ingests sugar, they end up feeling, at the very least, bloated and uncomfortable.

The low-FODMAP diet has been around since 2001, but it has taken some time to gather evidence to support the benefits of the diet. Over time, though, an increasing number of individuals have gotten relief from their IBS symptoms by cutting out high-FODMAP foods. Individuals with other conditions have also found it helpful.

My GI doc recommended this diet as a solution to my IBS. It has made a huge difference. We also did some testing and I know now that I cannot digest sugar properly. This diet is not hard to follow if you cook at home. I have found it challenging to eat at restaurants. But the longer I've been on this diet, the easier it is. I've not added much back to my diet yet. I just feel like I'm doing so well, I can stand to lose those foods. I can leave the house without feeling scared now. So it's worth it for me to continue to follow this diet.

—HALAH

WHAT TO EXPECT

Over the first four weeks, you will eliminate or minimize foods containing FODMAPs. During that time, you will track your

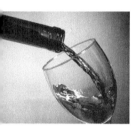

IBS symptoms so you can note improvements and determine how the plan is working for you.

After four weeks, you will strategically reintroduce foods into your diet to determine which ingredients trigger your IBS symptoms. By identifying food triggers, you can begin to customize your low-FODMAP diet plan to meet your own unique needs.

To ensure success you should also incorporate the following guidelines along with the low-FODMAP diet:

- Avoid caffeine, fats, and alcohol. These are not FODMAPs but can create serious issues in your digestive tract.
- Do not over eat. Keep your portions moderate.
- Savor your food. When eating quickly, you can gulp air, creating gas and bloating.
- Don't let your stomach get too empty. When you're excessively hungry, you might overindulge, especially if your blood sugar drops too fast.
- Eat in peace with no adrenaline-fueled discussions about work or stressful personal issues.

BENEFITS OF THE LOW-FODMAP DIET

The low-FODMAP diet is recognized as a potential management option for people suffering from IBS and other gastrointestinal disorders. FODMAPs are not unhealthy or reactive for many people; some can consume huge amounts of these foods with no issues, but when you are sensitive to FODMAPs you will receive some benefit when following the low-FODMAP diet. Some benefits associated with the low-FODMAP diet are:

Reduction or elimination of IBS symptoms This benefit is probably the most important for people with IBS. In clinical trials, over 75 percent of the IBS patients who participated reported a reduction of symptoms. Bloating, gas, constipation, diarrhea, and painful cramps diminished during the course of the research project. This diet is not a cure-all, and there is a range of improvement from complete disappearance of unpleasant digestion issues to no effect at all.

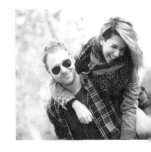

Improvement of mood Obviously if you have a happy stomach, you will probably feel more positive emotionally. This better mood might also have deeper roots in your body. There is a connection between lactose and fructose malabsorption and mild depression. People who have absorption issues have lower tryptophan concentrations in the body, and the tryptophan present is not absorbed well when there are high concentrations of fructose in the intestines. Tryptophan is an essential amino acid that is required to synthesize serotonin, a neurotransmitter associated with feeling good emotionally. Too little tryptophan can cause an imbalance in serotonin levels, creating mood imbalance that can lead to depression. A low-FODMAP diet (in particular, low-fructose intake) has been linked to an improvement in the symptoms of depression for some patients.

Understanding which foods cause issues The elimination diet associated with FODMAPs will help identify exactly which foods cause your IBS symptoms to worsen as well as foods which can be added back to your meals with no ill effects. This information is crucial when planning your meals so that you have no digestive issues.

Reset your food tolerance levels It might seem strange that after eliminating FODMAP foods that trigger your IBS symptoms, you can then add them back in with no ill effects or at least tolerate small amounts. Your body has a tolerance cutoff point for almost everything you eat. Have you even eaten several pints of strawberries because they are in season and felt awful afterward? If you eat FODMAP foods every day and have a low tolerance for them, even a little can send you into intestinal distress eventually. By completely eliminating these foods and allowing your system to reset, you can start fresh and keep your consumption under your personal tolerance level.

A cleaner healthier gut Gut health is crucial to general health and can be a contributing factor to autoimmune diseases and conditions such as IBS. Removing FODMAP foods can help rebalance your gut flora and calm inflammation caused by this food sensitivity. When your gut becomes healthier you will be able to eat FODMAP foods in small amounts again in some cases, and your digestion will improve universally.

? **When I read about FODMAPs, I get conflicting information about foods that are and are not considered low-FODMAP items. Why is that happening?** More and more foods are being evaluated for the quantity and type of FODMAPs they contain. Information is released as it becomes available, and sometimes it supports previous information, sometimes it contradicts it. In addition, people with IBS and similar conditions have to take a very personal approach to controlling what and how they eat. Books and websites based on personal experience with FODMAPs have some valuable information, but always regard online anecdotal statements with caution. A third consideration is that foods are not as uniform as you might imagine. One beet is quite different from another, so likewise, some people find a certain food tolerable on a low-FODMAP diet while others do not. Response can depend on factors like the variety that was grown, the soil it grew in, how old the vegetable was when you ate it, and how much of it you consumed.

What Is IBS?

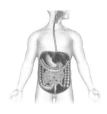 Irritable bowel syndrome (IBS) is a condition of the large intestine (colon or bowel) that can cause changes in bowel habits, pain, and gas. The cause of this disorder is not known, and it likely can be triggered by numerous factors, so treatment can vary depending on the severity of symptoms and individual sensitivities. Many people with IBS can control their symptoms by addressing lifestyle choices such as stress management and diet.

There is no definitive test to diagnose IBS, so it is important to consult your health care provider to discuss any symptoms and rule out other conditions. The symptoms of IBS can come and go and differ in both intensity and variety depending on each individual. Symptoms tend to worsen after meals and can include:

- Gas or bloating
- Constipation
- Cramping or abdominal pain
- Diarrhea
- Feeling of incomplete voiding during a bowel movement
- Heartburn after normal-size meals
- Low back ache
- Mucus in the stool

IBS symptoms do not include blood in your stool, unexplained weight loss, fever, vomiting, or increased urination, so if you also suffer from any of these symptoms, it is important to pursue other diagnoses to safeguard your health.

IT'S NOT JUST FOR IBS

While early studies showed the effectiveness of a low-FODMAP diet for IBS, research is now underway to test how low-FODMAP eating may affect other bowel health issues.

IBD

According to the Mayo Clinic, inflammatory bowel disease is an autoimmune condition involving inflammation of the digestive tract. The most common forms of IBD are Crohn's disease and

ulcerative colitis. The University of Virginia Medical Center notes that while more research is needed, primary results indicate that a low-FODMAP diet may also help manage symptoms associated with IBD.

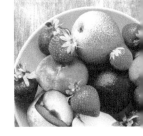

Fructose malabsorption

Fructose malabsorption is a condition in which the body poorly tolerates fructose intake. Researchers at the University of Austria found that fructose malabsorption may cause symptoms similar to those of IBS. Since the low-FODMAP diet is also low in fructose, it may be effective in minimizing symptoms associated with fructose intolerance. However, while the low-FODMAP diet is low in fructose, it is not fructose-free, so it is best to discuss this plan with your primary health care provider before adopting it to manage fructose malabsorption.

Celiac disease and gluten intolerance

Celiac disease is an inflammatory autoimmune disorder in which consumption of any foods containing gluten causes damage to the villi in the small intestine. This causes a number of intestinal issues, including gastrointestinal distress and an inability to digest foods and absorb nutrients.

According to the National Foundation for Celiac Awareness, about 1 in 133 Americans has celiac disease. The only treatment for celiac disease is a completely gluten-free diet. The low-FODMAP diet is not completely gluten-free, but it can easily be adapted to be so. Some low-FODMAP diets include a few gluten-containing ingredients such as oats (which is often processed in the same factories as wheat and barley) and asafetida powder, which is often used as a replacement for onions. Avoid these ingredients if you choose a low-FODMAP diet to manage celiac disease.

I have food allergies and sensitivities that already limit the foods I can safely eat. Will there be anything left to eat if I start a low-FODMAP diet?
The low-FODMAP diet is varied enough to adapt to such special concerns as milk or soy allergies, although the very early stages of the diet may seem a bit restrictive. Concentrate on foods you know you can eat without a problem, and focus on finding simple, safe ways to add more flavor and color to dishes through herbs and spices.

SIGNS OF DIGESTIVE DISORDER

If you haven't gotten a specific diagnosis for having a digestive disorder, you may still suspect that foods you are eating are making you sick. The reactions you have may be subtle but noticeable. Eventually, you can begin to anticipate them, since they happen every time you eat.

There are a lot of reasons you might be suffering— from food allergies and celiac disease to lactose intolerance or even food-borne illnesses. Talking to your doctor and getting tested is critical.

Learning to avoid foods that are to blame and to concentrate on foods that don't make you suffer is the goal of the low-FODMAP diet. If the following symptoms describe you, this may be a sign that FODMAPs are to blame:

- Mealtime makes you vaguely anxious, because you know that in a few minutes or hours, you will start to feel cramps, or worse.
- You feel uncomfortable when you are out in public because you just can't tell when you will need to find a bathroom.
- Your stomach pains are so strong you cannot concentrate on work.
- Whether you get plenty of sleep or not, you feel worn out and exhausted.
- You have heartburn after you eat. Maybe over-the-counter antacids work or maybe you feel like you need something stronger.

- You don't plan outings in the great outdoors because there are no bathrooms.
- You are losing weight, and you are not trying to.
- You describe yourself as having a "sensitive" stomach.
- Healthy foods like apples and onions make you feel uncomfortable, or worse.
- You can't remember the last time you felt like going to a restaurant; every time you go to one, you end up feeling sick.

People get used to the way they are and often just put up with it. When the symptoms continue to get worse, it only means that the condition has gone untreated for a long time, doing more and more damage to your stomach and cheating your body out of the nourishment it needs.

Any digestive disorder is a serious condition. If you suspect that you have one, it is important to know exactly what kind of disorder you have. Pains that occur an hour or two after meals or in the morning, for instance, and go away after eating food or taking an antacid are typical of ulcers. IBS doesn't cause a skin reaction or wheezing, but a food allergy might. Your specific condition may be one that requires a medical treatment, possibly in combination with a low-FODMAP diet. Here are nine common signs of a digestive disorder to discuss with your doctor:

1. Persistent abdominal pain and cramps
2. Diarrhea
3. Fever
4. Blood in the stool
5. Bloating
6. Constipation
7. Unexplained weight loss
8. Gas
9. Persistent heartburn

High-FODMAP Additives

When reading labels, look for the following ingredients, which may aggravate your IBS. While the following list is far from comprehensive, avoid foods that contain the following ingredients:

- Agave nectar
- Artificial flavorings
- Barley and any ingredient that contains the word (except barley malt vinegar or barley malt flavoring)
- Corn sugar
- Corn syrup
- Flour
- Flours made from legumes
- Fructose
- Fruit juice
- Herb and spice blends (may contain onion or garlic)
- High-fructose corn syrup (HFCS)
- Honey
- Inulin
- Rye and any ingredient that contains the word
- Semolina
- Sweeteners ending in -ol
- Wheat and any ingredient that contains the word

10 IBS TRIGGER FOODS

High-fat foods If you have IBS, you need to avoid fried foods, pizza, and fatty meats, because lots of fat will intensify intestinal contractions. It can also cause heartburn, because fatty foods can relax the valve that seals acid in the stomach, allowing it to rise into the esophagus. Fat is a very powerful gastrointestinal stimulant, which means it can produce indigestion and pain in people who have IBS.

Nuts The insoluble fiber in some nuts, cashews, or pistachios can make IBS symptoms worse because it stimulates the digestive system. Nuts and seeds can also be quite high in fat, which is also a trigger for IBS. Almonds, chia seeds, pecans, and pumpkin seeds are low-FODMAP and can be enjoyed in moderation.

Dairy You are considered to be lactose intolerant when your body cannot digest lactose, the sugar found in dairy products. This condition can cause cramps, diarrhea, and bloating. If you are not lactose intolerant, and still have issues with dairy, try non-fat or low-fat products because you could be reacting to the fat in milk or yogurt. You can also try dairy alternatives such as unsweetened almond milk or unsweetened rice milk.

Whole grains About 50 percent of people with IBS also suffer from gluten intolerance. Gluten is the protein found in whole grains like wheat, barley, or rye. If your body is sensitive to gluten, it can trigger your immune system to attack the cells of the small intestine, creating digestive upset and, in some cases, chronic disease. Even without an intolerance to gluten you might experience problems with your morning oatmeal because the insoluble fiber in whole grains can also cause diarrhea.

Vegetables Nutritious vegetables are often part of a healthy diet, but there are some that can create digestive issues. These troublesome vegetables include onions, cabbage, broccoli, beans, garlic, and red peppers. Raw produce in particular can cause issues due to the high insoluble fiber.

Sweeteners This category includes artificial sweeteners, honey, sugar substitutes, sugar-free foods, and many diet foods. Artificial sweeteners produce bloating and gas because they cannot be digested easily. The fructose that is found in honey and fruit can cause gas, bloating, and diarrhea. Fruit juices can be particularly high in fructose, so avoid drinking these if you feel they create digestive distress.

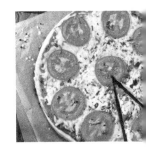

Beverages There are many different drinks that can cause issues when you have IBS. Beverages that are dehydrating such as coffee, carbonated drinks, and alcohol can contribute to constipation. Caffeinated beverages stimulate the production of acid in the stomach, causing heartburn and inflammation. The carbonated drinks can also create gas and bloating.

Spicy foods People with IBS can have nerve fibers in their intestines that react negatively to capsaicin, a substance in chili peppers that makes them hot. This reaction can cause pain. Many spicy foods are also fatty, such as chili, Mexican food, and some curries, which means that even foods without chili peppers can create digestive problems.

Beans Although they are a fabulous source of protein and fiber, beans can create serious digestive distress if you have IBS. Beans can help prevent constipation but the tradeoff may be cramps, gas, and bloating.

Chocolate Although packed with healthy antioxidants, chocolate can trigger IBS symptoms. It is a diuretic, which can produce constipation. Chocolate also contains caffeine, which can stimulate the intestines, causing painful inflammation and, in some cases, diarrhea.

> **"** I find the FODMAP diet offers a subtle and doable diet guide if you have bean or dairy sensitivities and helps with balancing out one's diet without drastically removing food groups or [taking] extreme measures nutritionally.
>
> **—ST. MICHELLE**

LOW-FODMAP DIET GUIDELINES

The key to relief of your symptoms is strictly following a low-FODMAP eating plan. Whenever you eat foods that contain FODMAPs, you may notice a return of unpleasant symptoms. The following guidelines can help you make the transition to low-FODMAP eating.

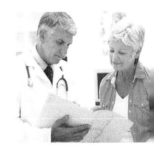

Talk to your doctor. Whenever you embark on a new eating plan, it is essential you meet with your primary health care provider. Talk to your doctor about getting screened for celiac disease before making plans to begin a low-FODMAP diet, since lowering your gluten intake with a low-FODMAP diet can make celiac testing inaccurate. If you have other serious food restrictions or health issues, such as a vegan diet or diabetes, it is especially important to seek medical advice before starting a low-FODMAP diet.

Follow the low-FODMAP diet strictly for four weeks, and track your progress. Let your symptoms be your guide. Track your progress using the symptom tracker on page XX. If after four weeks you still aren't feeling better, continue for two more. If your symptoms persist after six weeks of strict adherence to a low-FODMAP diet, it is time to talk to your physician and engage in a new strategy for symptom management.

After four to six weeks, begin reintroducing foods. After following the diet strictly for four to six weeks, slowly add FOD-MAP foods back into your diet to determine which foods trigger your IBS symptoms. Reintroduce foods one at a time, and only in a small amount. During this time, track your symptoms to determine which foods are your personal triggers. Note the food you've tried, the amount, and any symptoms you experienced as a result.

Read labels carefully. Food manufacturers sneak all kinds of ingredients into processed foods. Therefore, it's up to you to learn the label terms that indicate when a food contains ingredients that may cause a flare-up of your IBS. See page 25 for food additives to avoid.

Eat unprocessed or minimally processed foods. Because ingredient labels can be so tricky to navigate, one of the best ways to avoid accidentally ingesting something that causes a flare-up is to eat as many whole, unprocessed foods as possible. The more a food has been altered from its natural state, the more likely it is to contain ingredients that may cause you difficulty. For example, a whole tomato used to make spaghetti sauce is far less likely to contain ingredients that cause issues than spaghetti sauce from a jar. Select unprocessed foods (normally found around the perimeter of the grocery store), including animal protein, suitable low-FODMAP fruits and vegetables, nuts and seeds (excluding pistachios and cashews), and lactose-free dairy.

Make foods from scratch whenever possible. When you make your own food, you know exactly what goes into it. That isn't the case with processed foods, fast foods, and restaurant meals. If time is an issue, you can make several meals on the weekend and freeze or refrigerate them to have on hand all week. You can also double recipes to create leftovers for a second meal.

Plan meals and snacks. Careful planning can help you avoid accidentally eating foods that contain FODMAPs. Plan meals and snacks a week in advance, and compile a grocery list so you get all you need for the week in a single trip to the store. If you're traveling, take low-FODMAP foods with you.

Be prepared when dining out. If you are planning to eat at a restaurant, familiarize yourself with the menu items that fit within your low-FODMAP lifestyle before you go out to eat. Many restaurants list menus and nutrition information on their websites. See page 51 for more tips about dining out.

A good temporary plan for equalizing your system if you have Irritable Bowel Syndrome (IBS). Doctors are stating this is not a long-term plan for the average person. However, if you are having any difficulties in the digestive tract, this is an excellent way to alleviate the pain and determine if you do indeed have an issue that needs to be dealt with.

—CONNIE W.

SYMPTOM TRACKER

Before beginning the low-FODMAP diet, record your baseline symptoms (gas, constipation, diarrhea, bloating, abdominal pain, etc.) and their severity on a scale of 1 to 10, where 1 is no reaction.

SYMPTOM	SEVERITY

Follow the low-FODMAP diet for four to six weeks. Record your symptoms at the end of each week to track your progress.

TIME PERIOD	SYMPTOMS	SEVERITY
END OF WEEK 1		
END OF WEEK 2		
END OF WEEK 3		
END OF WEEK 4		
END OF WEEK 5		
END OF WEEK 6		

If your symptoms have improved dramatically, you can reintroduce foods containing FODMAPs back into your diet one at a time. Use the following table to track your body's reactions to each FODMAP food type.

FODMAP TYPE	FOOD AND SERVING SIZE	DATE/TIME OF EATING	SYMPTOMS	CONCLUSION

How to Reintroduce Foods

1 Select a food that contains only one type of FODMAP from one of the eliminated groups (fructans, polyols, fructose, lactose, or GOS). Avoid choosing foods like apples, which contain multiple FODMAPs. Otherwise, you won't know which FODMAP is triggering your symptoms.

2 Try a small amount. For example, if you've really missed wheat, try a half cup of pasta at lunch or dinner and note any symptoms that occur within the next 24 hours.

3 If you experience symptoms, chances are that food group is a trigger. For example, if you had a half cup of pasta and you noticed symptoms, then fructans are likely to be a trigger. You will need to restrict them.

4 After your symptoms disappear, try a smaller amount of the same food or move on to another food group.

5 If you don't experience symptoms, try the same food or a similar food from the same group in a slightly larger quantity. For example, you may wish to have one cup of pasta or two slices of bread.

6 Again, track your symptoms for 24 hours. If you remain symptom-free, you may continue to try the same FODMAP group, adding slightly larger quantities each day. If, after a week, you still haven't had symptoms, then you can assume this group is not a trigger and move on to the next.

HOW TO IDENTIFY TRIGGER FOODS

Trigger foods are those that cause flare-ups of your symptoms. You will most likely identify trigger foods once you have completed your initial four weeks of low-FODMAP eating and begin

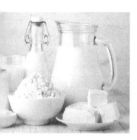

reintroducing foods into your diet. If you are not strictly following the low-FODMAP plan before you begin reintroducing foods, then you will not be able to assess your triggers accurately.

The low-FODMAP diet is a dynamic process. Even after you've gone through the full elimination and reintroduction, you may encounter other foods that trig-

ger your IBS. When you experience a flare-up of symptoms, use the following tips to identify the food or beverage that has triggered them.

- Track the foods you eat daily, even after the elimination and reintroduction phase of the diet.
- If you experience symptoms, check the foods you've eaten within eight hours of the start of symptoms. Look for unusual foods you don't eat regularly.
- Avoid all of those foods for one week.
- Once symptoms have subsided, reintroduce the potential trigger foods in small amounts, one at a time.
- Note which of these foods trigger a recurrence of symptoms and remove them from your diet.

ADAPTING THE LOW-FODMAP DIET

The low-FODMAP diet is meant to eliminate foods that can cause digestive distress and has very little wiggle room if you want a flexible diet. You can adapt the diet to include favorite recipes if you change the recipes to exclude FODMAPs, but to be successful, you can't deviate too far from the plan. You can still enjoy vegetarian foods, baked goods, smoothies, and even Paleo choices if those foods suit your needs, just carefully review ingredients in your recipes before eating them. You will find many delicious, nutritious foods in the low-FODMAP diet to suit your individual needs without leaving you feeling deprived. If you need to adapt the low-FODMAP diet to health conditions such as diabetes, your supervising dietician can ensure you are within compliance of your health needs.

Can I lose weight on the low-FODMAP diet? Some foods on the low-FODMAP diet are consumed in small quantities. This kind of portion awareness is a good start for weight loss. You can adjust serving sizes to keep calories under control, as long as you don't restrict yourself too severely. Be sure you are eating enough to maintain your overall health and energy levels. Many people report that they do lose weight on the low-FODMAP plan without planning to do so. Whether that is because they are simply paying more attention to what they eat or because the inflammation and water-retention in the gut diminishes is hard to establish.

How to Find a FODMAP Dietician

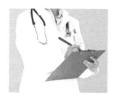 The low-FODMAP diet should be supervised by a registered dietician to ensure your plan is sound nutritionally. A dietitian is different than a nutritionist, so make sure you are consulting with the correct professional. Registered dietitians can give qualified advice on every aspect of eating and diet, including special diets, such as low-FODMAPs. This profession is regulated, and dietitians are professionally qualified through accredited learning institutions. Nutritionists are also qualified to give advice about healthy eating but usually cannot consult on special diets.

You can find a registered dietitian to assist with a low-FODMAP diet plan by asking your doctor or contacting the local hospital for a list. There are also many resources on the Internet if you search for dietitians in your area, and make sure you narrow the search to include only those familiar with low-FODMAP plans. Another great resource is the website IBSFree.net. You can click the Dietitian tab on the top and access "Find a Dietitian" in the drop-down menu. This will load a comprehensive spreadsheet showing approximately 160 dietitians, who might accept new clients needing assistance with FODMAPs. No matter where you find help to implement a low-FODMAP diet, make sure you independently verify the dietitian's credentials.

ALLERGIES VERSUS INTOLERANCES

Some people use the terms *food allergies* and *food intolerances* interchangeably. Medically, however, there is a difference between the two.

Food allergies cause an immediate immune system response in your body whenever you consume the item to which you are allergic. This immune response can affect many of your body's different organs, and symptoms are often 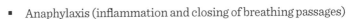 quite severe. This occurs when you consume even a tiny amount of the offending food. Allergic reactions include:

- Anaphylaxis (inflammation and closing of breathing passages)
- Difficulty breathing
- Drop in blood pressure
- Skin reactions such as hives
- Sudden onset of diarrhea, vomiting, or cramps
- Swelling or tingling of mouth, face, lips, throat, and tongue
- Upper respiratory symptoms
- Watery eyes

Food intolerances are much slower acting than allergies. Symptoms do not result from an immune system reaction. Instead, they typically come on gradually or may occur only when you eat a significant amount of the offending food. For example, in some cases, IBS results from FODMAP intolerances. Intolerances often manifest as gastrointestinal distress, although some may trigger asthma or other respiratory symptoms.

FODMAP FAQS

You've been given a lot of information, and you probably have questions. The following are the most commonly asked questions about low-FODMAP diets.

Q. How will I know if the low-FODMAP diet will work for me?
If you have IBS, studies have shown the diet is effective in about

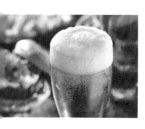

75 percent of cases when people strictly adhered to the dietary guidelines. Research is less clear about the diet's efficacy in cases of other bowel disorders, including IBD and celiac disease. After discussing it with your doctor, the best way to know for certain whether the diet will work for you is to try it. When you do, track your symptoms, and follow the guidelines exactly. If, after six weeks, you continue to have symptoms, the diet may not be right for you.

Q. Will I ever be able to go back to eating bread (or some other food I love)?
Maybe. While there's a good chance you'll have to follow some type of FODMAP restriction for the rest of your life, different people have varying FODMAP triggers. During the reintroduction phase, you'll discover your triggers. Foods that trigger symptoms will need to be avoided for a few months at least. But since tolerances to FODMAPs can change over time, you can reintroduce your favorite foods in small amounts again later to see if your tolerances have improved.

Q. *Can I enjoy a glass of wine, a beer, or a mixed drink on the low-FODMAP diet?*

WebMD notes that alcoholic beverages can trigger IBS symptoms. While most alcoholic beverages aren't high in FODMAPs, they can irritate your condition. You should be able to determine whether alcohol is one of your personal triggers by tracking symptoms. You may want to do this outside of your initial low-FODMAP diet and reintroduction of food so you don't confuse your results or misidentify a trigger.

Q. *What about coffee, tea, and soda?*

Black coffee doesn't contain FODMAPs, and black, green, and peppermint teas are low in FODMAPs. However, other teas like chamomile and oolong do contain FODMAPs, and sodas often have HFCS. Caffeine can stimulate bowel movements, which may be a problem for some people. When it comes to beverages, proceed with caution.

Q. *Is a low-FODMAP diet gluten-free?*

Wheat, barley, and rye are primary sources of gluten, and the diet restricts these. Some gluten-containing ingredients are allowed on the low-FODMAP diet, however. In a gluten-free diet for celiac disease, it is essential to avoid any wheat, barley, and rye and to avoid cross-contamination of these ingredients. Unless you also have celiac disease or some other form of gluten intolerance, it isn't necessary to be as strict about cross-contamination in a low-FODMAP diet.

Q. *Can I cheat?*

It is important to follow the plan strictly until you begin to reintroduce foods after the initial four weeks.

Q. *How can I get flavor into my food without using garlic and onions?*

There are several strategies you can use to flavor your foods. To replace onion and garlic flavor you can: Use the green part of scallions or leeks (but not the white part); Use a pinch of asafetida powder. If you have celiac disease, then you'll need to

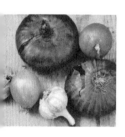

choose asafetida powder that is gluten-free; Make garlic oil by simmering garlic in oil, then removing all traces of the solid garlic (see page 92); Make onion oil by simmering onions in oil, then removing all traces of the solid onion.

Q. *Can I adapt a low-FODMAP diet?*

Yes, the low-FODMAP diet can be adapted to any eating plan. However, it is essential you talk with your doctor and/or work with a dietitian to ensure you are receiving proper nutrition.

Q. *I have diabetes. Can I be on a low-FODMAP diet?*

You can, although you will need to do a lot of adapting of the diet to meet your own dietary needs. One of the groups of foods restricted on the low-FODMAP diet is sugar alcohols, which are commonly used in sweet treats for diabetics. Before trying the low-FODMAP diet, talk with the health care provider and the dietitian managing your diabetes care.

Q. Will I get all the nutrients I need on a low-FODMAP diet?
The low-FODMAP diet can be a balanced diet depending on the foods you choose. For example, if you choose to eat only potato chips and candy bars to avoid FODMAPs, then the diet won't be balanced. However, if you choose foods from all food groups, then chances are you will get the nutrients you need. You can also work with a dietitian or physician to ensure you are eating a fully balanced and healthy diet.

The low-FODMAP Diet is designed for people plagued by digestive issues such as IBD (Inflammatory Bowel Disease) and IBS (Irritable Bowel Syndrome), Crohn's, GERD (acid reflux), and peptic ulcers. This diet recommends reducing the amount of foods that fall under the categories of fructans (e.g.,wheat), galactans (e.g.,legumes), lactose (e.g.,dairy products), fructose (e.g.,honey and some fruits), sugar alcohols (e.g.,stone fruits and cauliflower).
—ELLEN SUE SPICER-JACOBSON

SEVEN-DAY STARTER MEAL PLAN

This seven-day meal plan is your launch pad for starting the low-FODMAP diet! During this first week, it is essential you monitor your symptoms using the symptom tracker on page 32. While most people experience immediate relief within the first seven days, it may take much longer before you see the full effect.

The first week is essentially a "detox" week where your body rids itself of all of the FODMAPs you've been eating until now,

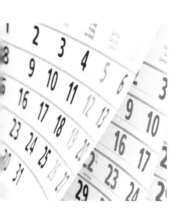

so you may notice some cravings for foods you cannot have. To fight cravings, plan to have a few low-FODMAP snacks and treats available. If you get a particularly intense craving, try engaging in an activity that releases endorphins into the brain, such as 10 minutes of exercise or meditation. The endorphins will help calm your food craving.

Your first week of meals includes breakfast, lunch, dinner with dessert, an afternoon snack, and an evening snack. Feel free to move snacks around as needed. To minimize waste and save time, meals and snacks use similar ingredients. Recipes included in this book are indicated with an asterisk (*).

Day One

Breakfast: Spiced Pumpkin Quinoa and Oat Cereal*
Lunch: Chicken Salad with Grapes*
Afternoon Snack: 2 cups Spiced Popcorn*
Dinner: Gluten-Free Penne with Basil-Walnut Pesto,* lettuce and tomato salad, Balsamic-Dijon Dressing,* Orange-Vanilla Smoothie*
Evening Snack: 2 cups Spiced Popcorn*

Day Two

Breakfast: Mixed Berry–Chia Breakfast Smoothie*
Lunch: Spinach, Strawberry, and Walnut Salad,* Balsamic-Dijon Dressing*
Afternoon Snack: 2 rice cakes, 2 tablespoons almond butter
Dinner: Steamed Clams, rice, steamed vegetables, Lemon-Rosemary Granita*
Evening Snack: Vanilla Chia Pudding with Blueberries*

Day Three

Breakfast: 2 hard-boiled eggs, ¾ cup honeydew melon
Lunch: deli rotisserie chicken on a bed of lettuce, Balsamic-Dijon Dressing*
Afternoon Snack: 1 (5-inch) celery stalk, 1 tablespoon almond butter
Dinner: Steak Fajitas with Bell Peppers* Lemon-Rosemary Granita*
Evening Snack: 2 cups Spiced Popcorn*

Day Four

Breakfast: crisp rice cereal, ½ sliced banana, ½ cup rice milk
Lunch: Strawberry, and Walnut Salad* ½ sliced banana
Afternoon Snack: ¾ cup honeydew melon cubes
Dinner: Balsamic-Dijon Grilled Chicken Skewers with Mixed Bell Peppers,* lettuce and tomato salad, Balsamic-Dijon Dressing,* Lemon-Rosemary Granita*
Evening Snack: 1 ounce Baked Corn Tortilla Chips,* ½ cup Baba Ghanoush*

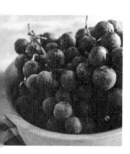

Day Five

Breakfast: ½ cup lactose-free plain yogurt, ½ cup halved grapes
Lunch: Deli rotisserie chicken, 1 cup rice, ¾ cup honeydew melon
Afternoon Snack: 10 baby carrots, 1 tablespoon almond butter or 2 tablespoons peanut butter
Dinner: hamburger patties on toasted gluten-free buns, Low-FODMAP Mayonnaise,* lettuce and tomato salad, Balsamic-Dijon Dressing,* Vanilla Chia Pudding with Blueberries*
Evening Snack: 1 ounce Baked Corn Tortilla Chips,* ½ cup Baba Ghanoush*

Day Six

Breakfast: Orange-Vanilla French Toast *
Lunch: Grilled Eggplant with Tomato and Basil Salad,*
sliced kiwi
Afternoon Snack: ½ cup halved grapes,
1 ounce peanuts
Dinner: Chicken Carbonara,* Lemon-Rosemary Granita*
Evening Snack: ½ cup halved grapes

Day Seven

Breakfast: Poached Eggs on Red Potato Hash*
Lunch: Chicken Salad with Grapes*
Afternoon Snack: 1 slice gluten-free toast, 2 tablespoons
peanut butter
Dinner: Balsamic-Dijon Grilled Chicken Skewers with Mixed
Bell Peppers,* Orange-Vanilla Smoothie*
Evening Snack: 1 ounce cheddar cheese, 2 rice cakes

TRICKS TO HELP YOU STAY ON TRACK

With a busy life, taking shortcuts is essential. The following tips and tricks can help you stay on track with your new low-FODMAP lifestyle:

Whenever possiblc, use precooked meats. This works especially well for salads and sandwiches, where cooking the meat in the same pan as the vegetables and other ingredients isn't essential for flavor development.

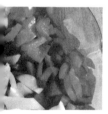

Choose chopped and washed vegetables. Use bagged salad, and chopped salad bar veggies to save time and effort.

Use instant rice. Regular rice takes 20 minutes or longer to cook. Instant rice is ready in 5 minutes. You can also purchase precooked rice in the freezer or rice section of the supermarket.

Parcook pasta. Cook pasta to 75 percent done, and then run it under cold water to stop cooking. Toss it with a bit of olive oil and store it in a tightly sealed container in the refrigerator until you're ready to use it (up to one week). Then cook it for the remaining 25 percent of the time in boiling water to serve.

Make stock on weekends. Many of the recipes in this book call for vegetable stock. You can double or triple the recipe to make a large pot so you only have to make it once or twice over the four weeks of the diet. Store it in 2- to 4-cup servings in the freezer and thaw it as necessary.

Low-FODMAP Diet for Children

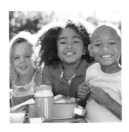

If your child has a definitive diagnosis of IBS, then it might be an appropriate to try a low-FODMAP diet with your doctor's approval. There is no current research on children and low-FODMAP diets, but clinical trials have shown no negative side effects in adults following the diet short-term. Long-term concerns about low-FODMAP diets include uncertain effects on gut flora and the risk of nutritional deficiencies. Discuss these issues with your child's doctor and follow these guidelines.

Involve your child: Explain the reasoning behind the low-FODMAP plan and the importance of sticking to it to feel better. Ask about substitutions for favorite foods and let your child help pick the menu.

Inform the people who need to know: Since your child's diet is going to change, it is important to let teachers, family members, babysitters, and parents of your child's friends know the situation.

Don't be too rigid: Children with FODMAP issues are not going to be in mortal danger if they eat these foods by accident; this is not like an extreme food allergy. Your child might eat something that has been eliminated and will have to go through whatever digestive issues that usually occur. Then continue with the diet without recriminations.

Be prepared: Always have low-FODMAP foods so that school lunches, snacks, and meals are easy and stress-free.

FOODS TO ENJOY AND AVOID

To help you make sense of which foods contain FODMAPs and which do not, the following table shows foods you need to eliminate and foods you can enjoy on a low-FODMAP diet. For foods that must be consumed in moderation, recommended serving sizes have been included.

Foods to Eliminate Moderation (High-FODMAP)	Foods to Enjoy (Low-FODMAP)	Foods to Enjoy in (Moderate-FODMAP)
FRUITS		
apples, apricots, avocados, blackberries, boysenberries, cherries, figs, fruit juice, lychees, mangos, nectarines, pears, persimmons, plums, prunes, watermelon	bananas, blueberries, cantaloupe ($^3/_4$ cup), clementines, cranberries, grapes, honeydew ($^3/_4$ cup), kiwis, lemons, limes, oranges, passion fruit, pineapples, raspberries, rhubarb, star fruit, strawberries	avocados (1 tablespoon), banana chips (10 chips), shredded coconut ($^1/_4$ cup), dried cranberries (1 tablespoon), grapefruit, pomegranate (1 small pomegranate or $^1/_4$ cup), raisins (1 tablespoon)
VEGETABLES		
asparagus, artichokes, beets, cauliflower, chicory, corn, garlic, scallions (white part), leeks (white part), mushrooms, okra, onions, peas, shallots, sugar snap peas	alfalfa sprouts, bean sprouts, bell peppers, bok choy, carrots, chiles, cucumbers, eggplant, endive, fennel, green beans, kale, leeks (green part), lettuce, olives, parsnips, potatoes, scallions (green part), spinach, summer squash, Swiss chard, turnips, zucchini	artichoke hearts ($^1/_8$ cup), broccoli ($^1/_2$ cup), Brussels sprouts, butternut squash ($^1/_4$ cup), celery (5-inch stalk), green cabbage (1 cup), radicchio (1 cup), savoy cabbage ($^1/_2$ cup), sweet potatoes ($^1/_2$ cup), tomato (1 tomato per meal)

Foods to Eliminate Moderation (High-FODMAP)	Foods to Enjoy (Low-FODMAP)	Foods to Enjoy in (Moderate-FODMAP)

STARCHES AND LEGUMES

barley, couscous, hummus, kidney beans, lima beans, pinto beans, rye, soybeans, wheat (and wheat-containing products, such as bread, cereal, crackers, flour, pasta, pretzels, tortillas, etc.)	arrowroot, gluten-free cornbread and corn tortillas, gluten-free breads, gluten-free flour, gluten-free pasta, millet, quinoa, rice, tapioca, tofu, tempeh	Buckwheat kernels ($1/8$ cup), canned chickpeas ($1/4$ cup), gluten-free oats ($1/4$ cup dry or $1/2$ cup cooked), canned lentils ($1/4$ cup), sourdough spelt bread (2 slices)

DAIRY

buttermilk, cottage cheese, custard, ice cream, milk (cow, goat, sheep), pudding, sour cream, most soy milks, yogurt	butter, coconut milk, lactose-free cow's milk, rice milk, whipped cream ($1/2$ cup)	Brie cheese, feta cheese, mozzarella cheese, hard cheeses (such as Parmesan, cheddar, and Swiss) (1 ounce); half-and-half ($1/4$ cup); soft cheeses (such as ricotta and cream cheese) (2 tablespoons)

NUTS AND SPICES

cashews, pistachios	Brazil nuts, chia seeds, macadamia nuts, peanuts, peanut butter, pecans, pine nuts, sesame seeds, sunflower seeds, walnuts	almonds (10 nuts), flaxseed (1 tablespoon), hazelnuts (10 nuts)

MEATS

processed meats containing wheat, garlic, onion, or HFCS	beef, chicken, duck, eggs, fish, game meats, lamb, pork, seafood, tofu, turkey	

Foods to Eliminate Moderation (High-FODMAP)	Foods to Enjoy (Low-FODMAP)	Foods to Enjoy in (Moderate-FODMAP)
CONDIMENTS		
condiments containing wheat, garlic, onion, or HFCS (such as barbecue sauce, ketchup, mayonnaise, mustard, teriyaki sauce, tomato paste)	champagne vinegar, fish sauce, garlic-infused oil (recipe on page 220), lemon juice, lime juice, oils, oyster sauce, red wine vinegar, rice vinegar, sherry vinegar, gluten-free soy sauce (tamari), white wine vinegar	balsamic vinegar (1 tablespoon)
HERBS AND SPICES		
garlic powder or salt, onion powder or salt	basil, bay leaves, caraway, cayenne, chervil, chives, cilantro, coriander, dill, ginger, mint, mustard seed, oregano, paprika, parsley, pepper, red pepper flakes, rosemary, salt, thyme, turmeric	allspice (1 teaspoon), cinnamon (1 teaspoon), onion-free and garlic-free chili powder (1 teaspoon), cumin (1 teaspoon)
SWEETENERS		
agave, agave nectar, agave syrup, HFCS, honey, isomalt, mannitol, sorbitol, xylitol	acesulfame-potassium (acesulfame-k), aspartame, brown sugar, pure maple syrup (2 tablespoons), sucrose, granulated sugar, powdered sugar	

10 TIPS FOR EATING OUT

Dining out in restaurants can be stressful on a low-FODMAP eating plan. Fortunately, there's plenty you can do to ensure you don't irritate your IBS when you eat out.

Plan ahead. Most restaurants post their menus online. Many chain restaurants also list ingredients and nutritional information. If necessary, you can call the restaurant ahead of time to ask about their ingredients.

Tell the waiter your dietary restrictions. Often, waitstaff (and even the chef) will be willing to work with you if you have food restrictions. Tell your server what your restrictions are and ask for recommendations.

Ask questions about the menu. Don't be afraid to ask questions about the menu. If the server doesn't know what's in a dish, he or she can ask the chef.

Visit the restaurant during non-peak hours. Servers and chefs are typically much more willing and able to work with special dietary requests when they aren't slammed with other customers.

Order simple menu items. For example, you're less likely to encounter FODMAPs if you order a steak, steamed vegetables, and potatoes than you are if you order something that requires more work such as a soup, sauce, or risotto.

Don't assume a food is safe. Even if you've ordered something simple such as a steak and baked potato, you need to make sure it hasn't been cooked with common ingredients like onions or garlic. Ask before ordering, and then ask again when it is delivered to the table.

If your order is incorrect, don't be afraid to send it back. Learn how to politely assert your dietary needs. Being afraid to speak up could cost you.

If you order a salad, don't order it with dressing. Instead, ask for oil and vinegar on the side and combine them yourself.

Use a low-FODMAP smartphone app. These apps can help you double-check ingredients you are unsure about.

Order items a la carte. If there are no composed dishes that will suit your diet, order a few sides, a salad, or appetizers that will. By ordering a la carte, you can create a balanced meal that meets your dietary needs.

66

Many suffer from diarrhea, cramping, and bloating caused by irritable bowel syndrome, or IBS. The low-FODMAP plan will not only allow you to cope with IBS, but will also allow you to relieve many of the symptoms caused by IBS.

—ALAN MCLAIN

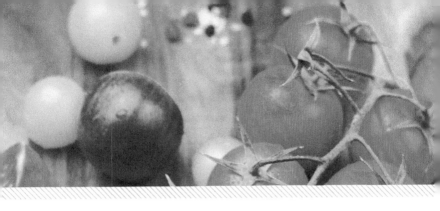

PART TWO

LOW-FODMAP DIET RECIPES

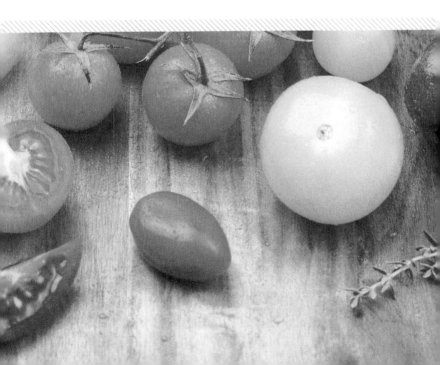

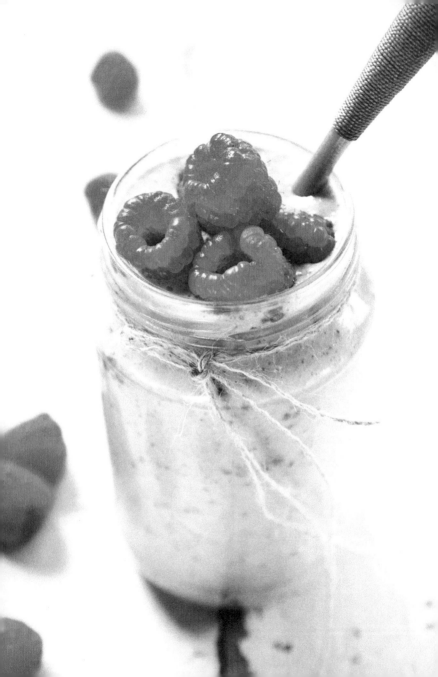

MIXED BERRY–CHIA BREAKFAST SMOOTHIE

NUT-FREE, VEGETARIAN, VEGAN, PALEO-FRIENDLY, DAIRY-FREE, SOY-FREE

Serves 2. Prep time: 5 minutes, plus 10 minutes to thicken. Cook time: None

Quick and easy for weekday mornings, this breakfast smoothie uses two types of berries. The smoothie is thickened with chia seeds, which also add protein. If fresh berries aren't available, you can use frozen berries instead, which will give the smoothie a thicker texture.

2 cups unsweetened rice milk

3 tablespoons chia seeds

1 cup sliced strawberries

1 cup raspberries

2 tablespoons pure maple syrup

1. In a liquid measuring cup, stir together the rice milk and chia seeds. Set aside, allowing the chia seeds to soak in the milk until the mixture thickens, about 10 minutes.

2. Stir the seeds and milk once more. Scrape the mixture into a blender jar. Add the strawberries, raspberries, and maple syrup.

3. Blend the smoothie on high until it is well combined, about 2 minutes. Serve.

Per Serving Calories 180; Protein 5g; Sugar 20g; Fat 7g

SPICED PUMPKIN QUINOA AND OAT CEREAL

VEGETARIAN, VEGAN, DAIRY-FREE, SOY-FREE

Serves 4. Prep time: 5 minutes. Cook time: 20 minutes

This spiced pumpkin cereal provides a warm start to the day. Oatmeal is high in fiber, while pumpkin provides additional fiber and vitamins A and C. When serving, offer lactose-free milk and brown sugar for those wishing a creamier or sweeter cereal.

1 cup unsweetened
   pumpkin puree

4 cups water

Pinch sea salt

¾ teaspoon ground cinnamon

1 cup quick oats

1 cup quinoa, rinsed

½ cup walnut pieces

1. In a large saucepan over medium-high heat, stir together the pumpkin, water, salt, and cinnamon and bring to a boil, stirring frequently. Add the oats and quinoa.

2. Reduce the heat to medium and cook, stirring frequently, until the oats and quinoa are cooked, about 15 minutes.

3. Remove the cereal from the heat and stir in the walnuts. Serve immediately.

Per Serving Calories 278; Protein 9g; Sugar 6g; Fat 11g

ORANGE-VANILLA FRENCH TOAST

NUT-FREE, VEGETARIAN

Serves 4. Prep time: 5 minutes. Cook time: 10 minutes

French toast is a family favorite. This low-FODMAP French toast uses lactose-free milk in place of cream and gluten-free bread. Serve with maple syrup on the side, if desired.

2 cups lactose-free whole milk

6 large eggs

Juice and grated zest of
    1 orange

1 teaspoon pure vanilla extract

8 slices gluten-free
    sandwich bread

2 tablespoons unsalted butter

Ground nutmeg, for garnish

1. In a medium-size bowl, whisk the milk, eggs, orange juice and zest, and vanilla extract until smooth. Pour the mixture into a 9-by-13-inch baking dish.

2. Preheat a nonstick skillet to medium-high.

3. Working in batches, soak the bread in the custard mixture until it is saturated.

4. Melt the butter in the skillet, coating the entire cooking surface. Place the soaked bread in the skillet and cook until browned on both sides, about 4 minutes per side.

5. Sprinkle the French toast lightly with nutmeg. Serve immediately.

Per Serving Calories 324; Protein 15g; Sugar 10g; Fat 12g

POACHED EGGS ON RED POTATO HASH

NUT-FREE, VEGETARIAN, PALEO-FRIENDLY, DAIRY-FREE, SOY-FREE

Serves 4. Prep time: 10 minutes. Cook time: 15 minutes

A ¼-inch dice on the red potatoes allows this hash to cook quickly. If you have a mandoline slicer, this will allow you to cut the potatoes evenly and quickly, although you can also use a knife. Keep the skin on the potatoes, as it adds fiber and flavor.

2 tablespoons Garlic Oil (page 92)

4 medium red potatoes, cut into ¼-inch dice

½ teaspoon sea salt

¼ teaspoon freshly ground black pepper

1 teaspoon white vinegar

4 large eggs

¼ cup chopped fresh chives

1. In a large sauté pan, heat the garlic oil over medium-high heat until it is shimmering. Add the potatoes to the pan. Season them with the salt and pepper. Cook, stirring frequently, until the potatoes are soft and well browned, about 10 minutes.

2. While the potatoes cook, fill a large saucepan with about 3 inches of water and bring to a simmer over medium heat. Add the vinegar to the simmering water. ▶

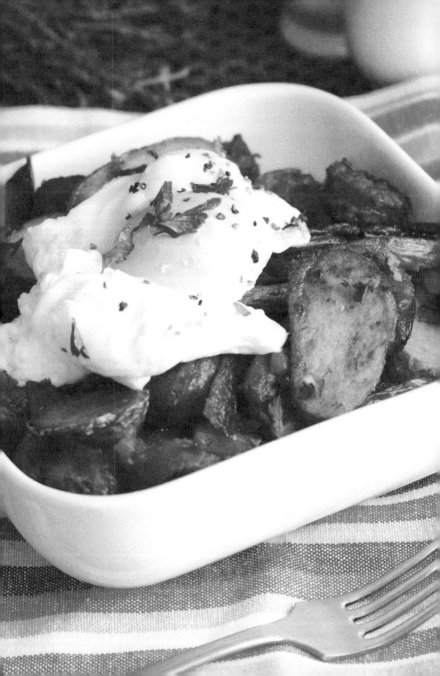

3. Crack 1 egg into a custard cup and carefully slip the egg into the simmering water. Repeat with each egg. Allow the eggs to simmer until the whites are set, about 4 minutes.

4. Divide the potatoes among four plates. Top the potatoes with the poached eggs. Sprinkle the chives evenly over the eggs, and serve.

Per Serving Calories 286; Protein 9g; Sugar 1.5g; Fat 9g

CHICKEN SALAD WITH GRAPES

PALEO-FRIENDLY, DAIRY-FREE, SOY-FREE

Serves 4. Prep time: 10 minutes. Cook time: None

This salad is a play on the classic Waldorf salad. Waldorf salads contain apples, which contain FODMAPs, so this salad replaces the apples with grapes. It is topped with a creamy dressing. Although the recipe specifies green grapes, you can choose any type of seedless grapes you wish.

12 ounces boneless, skinless chicken breast, grilled and cut into ½-inch cubes

2 celery stalks, chopped

½ cup chopped fennel

1 cup halved green grapes

½ cup chopped walnuts

1 cup Low-FODMAP Mayonnaise (page 89)

½ teaspoon sea salt

½ teaspoon freshly ground black pepper

4 large butter lettuce leaves

1. In a large bowl, toss together the chicken, celery, fennel, green grapes, and walnuts until well combined.

2. Add the mayonnaise, salt, and pepper. Toss again to combine.

3. Serve the salad in the butter lettuce leaves.

Per Serving Calories 507; Protein 29g; Sugar 8g; Fat 35g

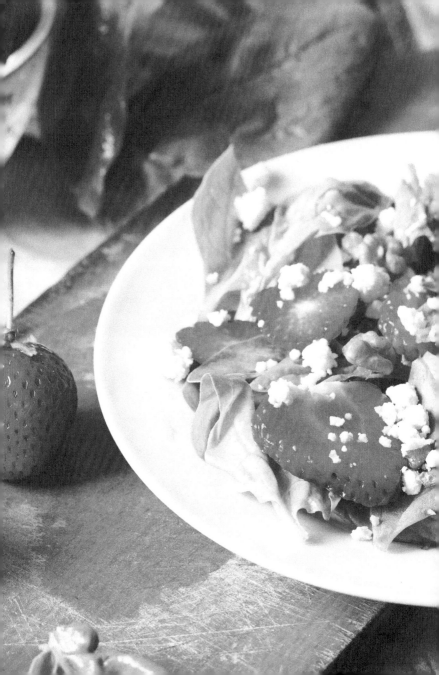

SPINACH, STRAWBERRY, AND WALNUT SALAD

VEGETARIAN, SOY-FREE

Serves 2. Prep time: 5 minutes. Cook time: None

Sliced red strawberries and bright green spinach make this a very pretty salad. If you take it to lunch, pack the salad separately from the vinaigrette and toss it with the vinaigrette just before eating. The Balsamic-Dijon Dressing on page 90 is the perfect accompaniment for the salad.

1 (9-ounce) bag baby spinach

1 cup sliced strawberries

1 ounce Parmesan cheese, shaved

½ cup walnut pieces

Freshly ground black pepper

¼ cup Balsamic-Dijon Dressing (page 90)

1. In a large bowl, combine the baby spinach, strawberries, cheese, and walnuts.

2. Grind pepper over the top. Add the vinaigrette and toss to combine. Serve.

Per Serving Calories 409; Protein 13g; Sugar 4g; Fat 27g

GRILLED EGGPLANT WITH TOMATO AND BASIL SALAD

NUT-FREE, VEGETARIAN, SOY-FREE

Serves 4. Prep time: 20 minutes, plus 1 hour to rest. Cook time: 10 minutes

Salting eggplant and allowing it to sit before you cook it draws out the water in the eggplant. This removes the bitterness and allows the eggplant to grill quickly. Wipe the salt off the eggplant, and pat it dry thoroughly with paper towels before putting it on the grill. You can also cook the eggplant in a sauté pan over medium-high heat for about 4 minutes per side if you don't have a grill.

For the garlic-basil vinaigrette

¾ cup Garlic Oil (page 92)

¼ cup red wine vinegar

2 tablespoons finely chopped fresh basil

¼ teaspoon sea salt

⅛ teaspoons freshly ground black pepper

For the eggplant and tomato salad

1 large eggplant, peeled and sliced crosswise into ¼-inch-thick slices

Sea salt

2 large heirloom or beefsteak tomatoes, seeded and diced

8 ounces mozzarella, cubed

Freshly ground black pepper

To make the garlic-basil vinaigrette

1. Whisk together the garlic oil, vinegar, basil, salt, and pepper in a small bowl.

2. Serve immediately, or store in a tightly sealed container in the refrigerator for up to 1 week.

To make the eggplant and tomato salad

1. Line a baking sheet with paper towels, and place the eggplant slices in a single layer on the paper towels. Sprinkle the eggplant with salt. Allow the salted eggplant to sit for 1 hour.

2. In a medium bowl, combine the tomatoes, mozzarella, and ½ cup of the vinaigrette. Set it aside to marinate while the eggplant rests.

3. Preheat the grill to high.

4. Lightly brush the grill grate with oil.

5. Wipe the salt from the eggplant and pat dry with paper towels.

6. Grill the eggplant slices over direct heat for 4 minutes per side.

7. Serve the eggplant warm, topped with the tomato salad. Season with pepper.

Per Serving Calories 521; Protein 17g; Sugar 5g; Fat 45g

BALSAMIC-DIJON GRILLED CHICKEN SKEWERS WITH MIXED BELL PEPPERS

NUT-FREE, PALEO-FRIENDLY, DAIRY-FREE, SOY-FREE

Serves 4. Prep time: 15 minutes, plus at least 1 hour to marinate. Cook time: 15 minutes

If you have time, marinate the chicken for the full 3 hours for the best flavor penetration. If you're running short on time, 1 hour will be adequate to impart flavor. If you don't have a grill, you can bake the skewers on a rimmed baking sheet in a 425°F oven for 8 to 10 minutes.

1 pound boneless, skinless chicken breasts, cut into 1-inch cubes

1 cup Balsamic-Dijon Dressing (page 90)

1 green bell pepper, seeded and cut into 1½ inch pieces

1 red bell pepper, seeded and cut into 1½ inch pieces

1 orange bell pepper, seeded and cut into 1½ inch pieces

1. Place the chicken in a large zipper-top plastic bag. Pour in ¾ cup of the dressing. Seal the bag and shake it to distribute the dressing. Place the bag in the refrigerator and allow it to marinate for 1 to 3 hours.

2. Heat the grill to high. ▶

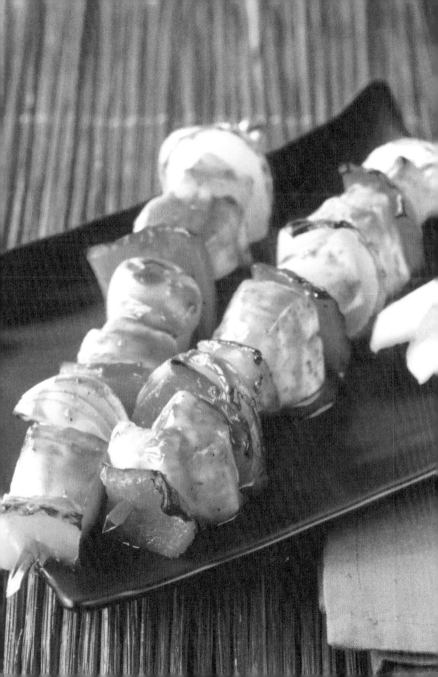

3. Lightly brush the grill grate with oil.

4. Thread the chicken and green, red, and orange bell peppers
    onto the skewers, alternating the chicken and the three
    colors of pepper.

5. Grill the skewers over direct heat, brushing the chicken and
    peppers with the remaining ¼ cup dressing. Cook, turning
    the skewers occasionally, until the chicken juices run clear,
    about 15 minutes. Serve.

Per Serving Calories 404; Protein 33g; Sugar 4g; Fat 27g

You can vary this recipe in many ways. For example,
replace the chicken with cubes of beef, pork, or lamb.
Mix with the marinade in the morning, and leave it
in the refrigerator all night. You can also use zucchini
cut into 1-inch cubes in addition to, or in place of, the
peppers.

ENCHILADAS WITH OLIVES AND CHEDDAR

NUT-FREE, VEGETARIAN, SOY-FREE

Serves 4. Prep time: 10 minutes. Cook time: 30 minutes

These enchiladas have a flavorful filling made from cheese, olives, and jalapeños. The enchilada sauce comes together quickly, because aromatic ingredients are pulsed together in a food processor into a very fine dice and then cooked quickly in olive oil. If you don't have a food processor, you can finely mince the vegetables with a knife. Be sure to choose a tomato sauce and a chili powder that do not have added garlic or onion.

For the enchilada sauce

6 scallions (green parts only)

1 jalapeño pepper, seeded

1 tablespoon chopped chives

3 tablespoons Garlic Oil (page 92)

1 (8-ounce) can tomato sauce

3 tablespoons chili powder

½ teaspoon dried oregano

½ teaspoon ground cumin

½ teaspoon sea salt

¼ teaspoon cayenne pepper

For the enchiladas

2 (4-ounce) cans chopped black olives, drained

1 (4-ounce) can diced jalapeño peppers, drained

8 ounces cheddar cheese, grated

8 (6-inch) corn tortillas ▶

To make the enchilada sauce

1. Place the scallion greens, fresh jalapeño, and chives in a food processor, and pulse briefly to mince the vegetables.

2. In a medium-size saucepan, heat the garlic oil over medium-high heat until it shimmers. Add the vegetables from the food processor and cook until very fragrant, about 2 minutes.

3. Add the tomato sauce, chili powder, oregano, cumin, salt, and cayenne. Simmer for 5 minutes to integrate the flavors, then remove from heat and set aside.

To make the enchiladas

1. Preheat the oven to 350°F.

2. In a small bowl, combine the olives, canned jalapeños, and 6 ounces of the cheese.

3. Dip each corn tortilla in the enchilada sauce. Spoon an equal portion of the cheese mixture down the center of each tortilla and roll them up. Place the rolled enchiladas in a 9-by-13-inch baking pan.

4. Pour the remaining sauce over the top of the enchiladas. Sprinkle with the remaining 2 ounces of cheese.

5. Bake the enchiladas until they are warm and bubbly, about 20 minutes. Serve.

Per Serving Calories 506; Protein 18g; Sugar 2g; Fat 36g

GLUTEN-FREE PENNE WITH BASIL-WALNUT PESTO

VEGETARIAN, SOY-FREE

Serves 4. Prep time: 5 minutes. Cook time: 10 minutes

Traditional pesto is a mixture of pine nuts, basil, Parmesan cheese, garlic, and olive oil. This pesto replaces the garlic with garlic oil and the pine nuts with walnuts. If you'd prefer a more traditional pesto, you can use an equal amount of pine nuts in place of the walnuts.

1 pound gluten-free penne pasta

2 cups tightly packed basil leaves

½ cup chopped walnuts

½ cup grated Parmesan cheese

⅓ cup Garlic Oil (page 92)

1. Bring a large pot of water to a boil over high heat. Add the penne and cook according to the package instructions until al dente, 9 to 11 minutes.

2. Meanwhile, pulse the basil, walnuts, Parmesan, and garlic oil in a food processor to finely chop and blend the ingredients. Do not puree.

3. When the pasta is done, drain it in a colander. Toss the hot pasta with the pesto. Serve immediately.

Per Serving Calories 727; Protein 22g; Sugar 2g; Fat 33g

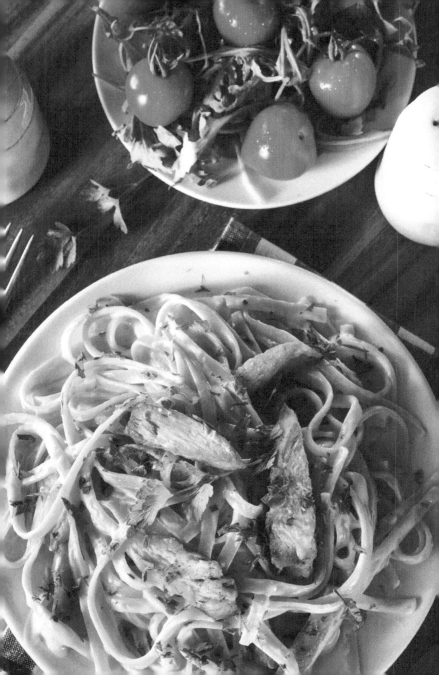

CHICKEN CARBONARA

NUT-FREE, SOY-FREE

Serves 4. Prep time: 10 minutes. Cook time: 30 minutes

Carbonara is a traditional Italian pasta with a bacon and egg sauce. This recipe includes chicken for extra protein. You can make the sauce while the spaghetti cooks, and then toss it with the hot, drained spaghetti so it coats every strand.

7 ounces gluten-free spaghetti

8 bacon slices, cut into
    ½-inch pieces

1 tablespoon Garlic Oil
    (page 92)

12 ounces boneless, skinless
    chicken breast, cut into
    1-inch pieces

6 scallions (green part only),
    chopped

3 eggs

¼ cup lactose-free whole milk

½ cup grated Parmesan cheese

Freshly ground black pepper

1. Bring a large pot of water to a boil over high heat. Cook the spaghetti according to the package directions until it is al dente, 8 to 12 minutes. Drain the pasta in a colander.

2. In a large sauté pan, cook the bacon over medium-high heat, stirring occasionally, until it is browned and crisp, about 5 minutes. ▶

3. Remove the bacon from the pan with a slotted spoon, and set it aside to drain on paper towels. Remove all but 1 tablespoon of the bacon fat from the pan and return the pan to the heat. Add the garlic oil and heat until it shimmers.

4. Add the chicken to the pan and cook, stirring occasionally, until it is completely browned on all sides, about 3 minutes per side. Remove the chicken from the pan with tongs and set it aside with the bacon.

5. Add the scallion greens to the pan and cook, stirring occasionally, until softened, about 4 minutes.

6. Meanwhile, in a small bowl, whisk together the eggs and milk until very well combined.

7. Add the hot spaghetti, bacon, and chicken to the pan with the scallion greens, and remove the pan from the heat.

8. Add the egg-milk mixture to the hot pasta in a thin stream, stirring constantly. Toss with the Parmesan cheese and pepper. Serve.

Per Serving Calories 650; Protein 50g; Sugar 1g; Fat 31g

 This recipe uses raw eggs, although the hot pasta cooks them slightly. To protect yourself from contamination from raw eggs, use very fresh eggs that are less than a week old or use pasteurized eggs.

STEAK FAJITAS WITH BELL PEPPERS

NUT-FREE, DAIRY-FREE, SOY-FREE

Serves 4. Prep time: 10 minutes, plus at least 1 hour to marinate.
Cook time: 15 minutes

For the most flavorful results, prepare the marinade the night before you make these fajitas and marinate the meat overnight in a zipper-top plastic bag. You can also marinate the beef for a shorter time, as little as 1 hour, although it won't be as flavorful.

¼ cup chopped fresh cilantro

3 scallions (green part only), minced

½ jalapeño pepper, seeded

½ teaspoon ground cumin

Juice of 1 lime

3 tablespoons Garlic Oil (page 92)

1 pound flank steak

8 (6-inch) corn tortillas

2 green bell peppers, seeded and sliced

2 yellow bell peppers, seeded and sliced

1. In a food processor, pulse the cilantro, scallion greens, jalapeño, cumin, lime juice, and 2 tablespoons of the garlic oil until minced and combined but not pureed. You can also finely mince the cilantro, scallion greens, and jalapeño with a knife if you don't have a food processor, and then whisk in the cumin, lime juice, and 2 tablespoons of the garlic oil. ▶

2. Place the flank steak in a zipper-top plastic bag and add the marinade. Seal the bag and push the steak around to coat it evenly. Place in the refrigerator to marinate for at least 1 hour, or overnight.

3. Preheat the oven to 350°F.

4. Wrap the corn tortillas in foil and warm them in the oven for 15 minutes.

5. Meanwhile, in a large sauté pan, heat the remaining 1 tablespoon of garlic oil over medium-high heat until it shimmers. Add the flank steak and cook until it is browned on the outside and medium-rare in the center, 3 to 4 minutes per side. Remove the steak from pan and set it aside, tented with foil.

6. Add the green and yellow bell peppers to the pan, and cook, stirring occasionally, until they are softened and brown, 5 to 6 minutes.

7. Slice the meat against the grain into ¼-inch-thick slices. Serve the meat wrapped in corn tortillas with the peppers.

Per Serving Calories 453; Protein 36g; Sugar 6g; Fat 21g

VANILLA CHIA PUDDING WITH BLUEBERRIES

NUT-FREE, VEGETARIAN, VEGAN, DAIRY-FREE, SOY-FREE

Serves 4. Prep time: 5 minutes, plus overnight refrigeration.
Cook time: None

Chia pudding makes a good snack because it is quick and very easy to make. It is also filling. When chia seeds soak in liquid, they swell and turn into a gel with a texture similar to tapioca. Top this pudding with fresh blueberries or any other low-FODMAP fruit.

2 cups unsweetened rice milk

¼ cup sugar

½ teaspoon pure vanilla extract

⅔ cups chia seeds

1 cup fresh blueberries

1. In a medium-size bowl, whisk together the rice milk, sugar, and vanilla until well combined.

2. Stir in the chia seeds. Allow the mixture to sit on the counter for 30 minutes. Then cover and refrigerate it overnight.

3. Before serving, stir in the blueberries.

Per Serving Calories 169; Protein 5g; Sugar 16g; Fat 8g

ORANGE-VANILLA SMOOTHIE

NUT-FREE, VEGETARIAN, SOY-FREE

Serves 4. Prep time: 5 minutes, plus 20 minutes to thicken.
Cook time: None

This delicious dessert smoothie has a delightful creamy orange flavor. If you'd like a more intense orange flavor, add 1 teaspoon of freshly grated orange zest. Use freshly squeezed orange juice for this recipe.

1 cup freshly squeezed
   orange juice
¼ cup chia seeds
2 cups lactose-free plain yogurt

1 cup lactose-free whole milk
¼ cup sugar
2 teaspoons pure vanilla extract
1 cup crushed ice

1. In a small bowl, combine the orange juice and chia seeds. Allow the mixture to sit for 20 minutes for the chia seeds to thicken and expand.

2. In a blender, combine the orange juice–chia mixture, yogurt, milk, sugar, vanilla, and crushed ice. Blend on high until smooth. Serve.

Per Serving Calories 355; Protein 16g; Sugar 30g; Fat 13g

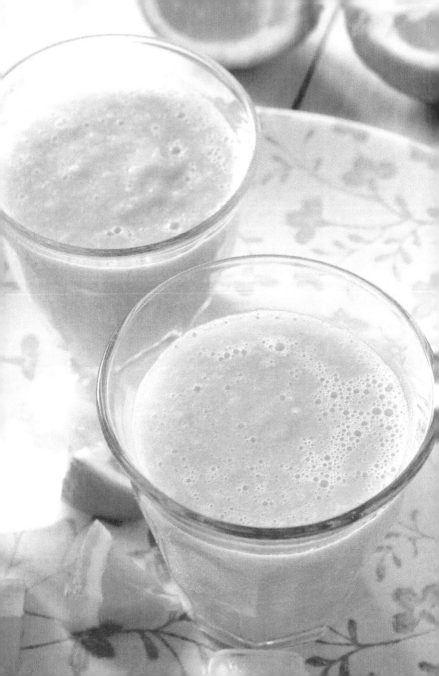

LEMON-ROSEMARY GRANITA

NUT-FREE, VEGETARIAN, VEGAN, DAIRY-FREE, SOY-FREE

Serves 4. Prep time: 10 minutes, plus 1 hour to freeze.
Cook time: 10 minutes

This granita is a sweet treat with just a hint of savory. If you can, select Meyer lemons, since they are juicier and slightly sweeter than regular lemons and have a more pronounced lemon flavor. The rosemary complements the lemon perfectly—be sure to use fresh rosemary, not dried. The granita will need several cycles of freezing and stirring to give it the right texture, but most of the time spent is just waiting for it to freeze.

3 cups water	Zest of 1 lemon
1 cup plus 2 tablespoons sugar	Juice of 6 lemons
5 rosemary sprigs	

1. In a medium saucepan over medium-high heat, bring the water, sugar, rosemary, and lemon zest to a simmer. Simmer, stirring constantly, until the sugar dissolves.

2. Remove the pan from the heat, cover, and allow the mixture to steep for 10 minutes.

3. Strain the syrup through a fine-mesh sieve into a large bowl and stir in the lemon juice. Whisk to combine.

4. Cover and chill the mixture in the refrigerator until cold, about 15 minutes.

5. Pour the chilled mixture into two 9-by-9-inch shallow
    baking pans and freeze. After 15 minutes, stir the granita
    with a large fork. Continue stirring and freezing in
    15-minute increments until the granita is completely frozen,
    about 1 hour. Serve.

Per Serving Calories 232; Protein 1g; Sugar 58g; Fat 1g

SPICED POPCORN

NUT-FREE, VEGETARIAN, SOY-FREE

Serves 4. Prep time: 5 minutes. Cook time: 5 minutes

Popcorn makes a great snack, but this popcorn is special because it's tossed with sweet and savory spices. Avoid microwavable popcorn since it may contain additives that aggravate IBS.

2 tablespoons canola oil

½ cup popcorn kernels

¼ cup unsalted butter, melted

½ teaspoon cayenne pepper

½ teaspoon ground cumin

½ teaspoon ground cinnamon

2 tablespoons brown sugar

1. Heat the canola oil in a heavy pot over high heat until it shimmers.

2. Add 1 kernel of popcorn and wait for it to pop. When the kernel pops, add the remaining popcorn and cover the pot.

3. Carefully shift the pot back and forth while maintaining contact with the stove top to stir the kernels. Cook until the popping slows to about 1 pop per second. Pour the popcorn into a large bowl.

4. In a small bowl, mix the melted butter, cayenne, cumin, cinnamon, and brown sugar. Pour the mixture over the popcorn. Serve immediately.

Per Serving Calories 183; Protein 0g; Sugar 4g; Fat 19g

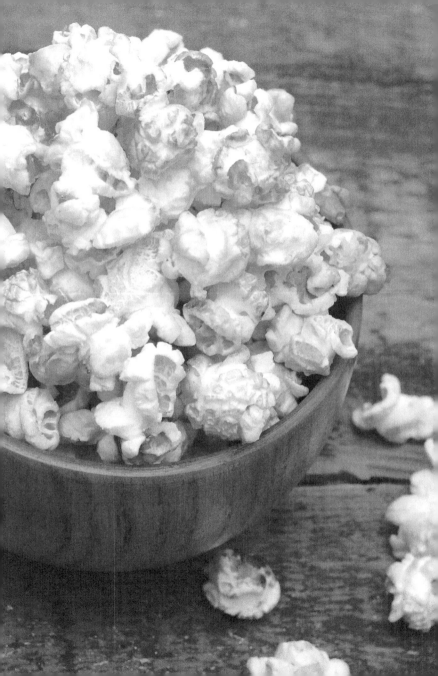

FRESH SALSA AND BAKED TORTILLA CHIPS

NUT-FREE, VEGETARIAN, VEGAN, DAIRY-FREE, SOY-FREE

Serves 4. Prep time: 15 minutes, plus 20 minutes to rest.
Cook time: 25 minutes

Commercially prepared salsa contains onions and garlic. This low-FODMAP version uses garlic oil and scallion greens to replace those flavors. This is an uncooked salsa, so it needs to be used within about 4 days of making it. Keep it tightly sealed in the refrigerator until you are ready to use it. Store the chips for up to 1 week in a tightly sealed container.

For the salsa

4 heirloom or beefsteak tomatoes, chopped

8 scallions (green part only), minced

¼ cup chopped fresh cilantro

2 tablespoons chopped fresh chives

1 jalapeño pepper, seeded and minced

Juice of 1 lime

1 tablespoon Garlic Oil (page 92)

½ teaspoon sea salt

½ teaspoon freshly ground black pepper

Pinch cayenne pepper

For the chips

12 (6-inch) corn tortillas

2 tablespoons olive oil

Sea salt (optional)

To make the salsa

1. In a medium bowl, toss together the tomatoes, scallions, cilantro, chives, jalapeño, lime juice, garlic oil, salt, black pepper, and cayenne until well mixed.

2. Allow the salsa to rest for 20 minutes before serving to blend the flavors.

To make the chips

1. Preheat the oven to 350°F.

2. Slice the tortillas into six triangles each, and place them in a large bowl. Add the olive oil and sea salt (if using) and toss to coat.

3. Place the coated tortilla chips in a single layer on two baking sheets. Bake until the chips are browned and crisp, 20 to 25 minutes.

Per Serving Calories 280; Protein 6g; Sugar 5g; Fat 8g

 Limit these to about 18 chips per day; any more may cause IBS upset.

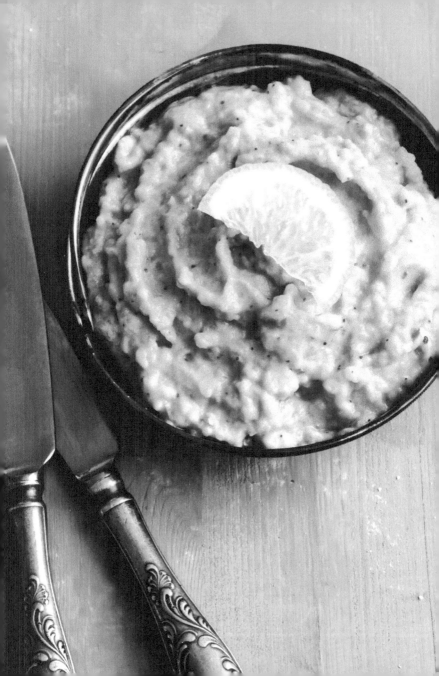

BABA GHANOUSH

NUT-FREE, VEGETARIAN, VEGAN, PALEO-FRIENDLY, DAIRY-FREE, SOY-FREE

Serves 4. Prep time: 15 minutes, plus 5 minutes to cool.
Cook time: 10 minutes

This eggplant dip is a traditional Middle Eastern snack. Traditional baba ghanoush calls for lots of garlic, which is replaced here with garlic oil. The recipe also leaves out the tahini, which is high in FODMAPs. Limit intake to less than 1 cup per day. Leftovers can be stored in a tightly sealed container in the refrigerator for up to 3 days.

1 large eggplant, peeled and cut into ¼-inch-thick slices

2 tablespoons olive oil

¼ cup freshly squeezed lemon juice

¼ teaspoon ground cumin

¼ teaspoon sea salt

¼ cup Garlic Oil (page 92)

1 tablespoon chopped fresh flat-leaf parsley

1. Heat the grill to high.

2. Lightly brush the grill grate with oil.

3. Brush each slice of eggplant with olive oil and place it on the hot grill. Grill, flipping occasionally, until the slices are very soft and have grill marks, about 5 minutes per side.

4. Allow the eggplant to cool slightly, about 5 minutes. ▶

5. Place the eggplant in a medium bowl and mash it with a fork. Add the lemon juice, cumin, and salt. Mix well. Taste and add additional salt, if necessary.

6. Drizzle the eggplant with the garlic oil and sprinkle it with the chopped parsley. Serve.

Per Serving Calories 213; Protein 1g; Sugar 3g; Fat 21g

 If you don't have a grill, you can roast the eggplant in a 450°F oven. To do this, keep the eggplant whole and unpeeled, and prick it all over with a fork. Roast on a baking sheet until the eggplant is soft, about 20 minutes. Allow the eggplant to cool and then remove the skin. Proceed with the recipe as indicated.

LOW-FODMAP MAYONNAISE

NUT-FREE, VEGETARIAN, PALEO-FRIENDLY, DAIRY-FREE, SOY-FREE

Makes 1 cup. Prep time: 10 minutes. Cook time: None

Many brands of prepared mayonnaise contain high-fructose corn syrup (HFCS). Fortunately, mayonnaise is quite easy to make at home. The trick lies in adding the oil very slowly. If you don't have a food processor, you can whisk constantly instead, making sure you carefully pour the oil in a very thin stream.

1 large egg yolk

1 tablespoon red wine vinegar

2 teaspoons freshly squeezed
   lemon juice

½ teaspoon sea salt

1 cup canola oil, light olive oil,
   or other neutral oil

1. In a food processor, combine the egg yolk, vinegar, lemon juice, and sea salt.

2. With the food processor running, start adding the oil, one drop at a time, through the feed tube. After about 20 drops of oil, start adding the remaining oil in a very thin stream with the food processor still running.

3. Serve immediately, or store the mayonnaise in a tightly sealed container in the refrigerator for up to 1 week.

Per Serving (2 tablespoons) Calories 115; Protein 0g Sugar 0g; Fat 10g

BALSAMIC-DIJON DRESSING

NUT-FREE, VEGETARIAN, VEGAN, PALEO-FRIENDLY, DAIRY-FREE, SOY-FREE

Makes 1 cup. Prep time: 5 minutes. Cook time: None

Balsamic vinegar is low in FODMAPs, provided you limit yourself to 1 tablespoon. This salad dressing recipe uses a 3:1 vinaigrette ratio, so 2 tablespoons of dressing has less than 1 tablespoon of balsamic vinegar. Limit yourself to one 2-tablespoon serving per meal.

2 tablespoons balsamic vinegar

2 tablespoons Dijon mustard

¼ teaspoon sea salt

⅛ teaspoon freshly ground black pepper

¾ cup Garlic Oil (page 90)

1. In a small bowl, whisk together the vinegar, mustard, salt, and pepper until well combined. Add the oil in a thin stream, whisking to emulsify.

2. Serve immediately, or store in a tightly sealed container in the refrigerator for up to 1 week.

Per Serving (2 tablespoons): Calories 184; Protein 0g; Sugar 0g; Fat 21g

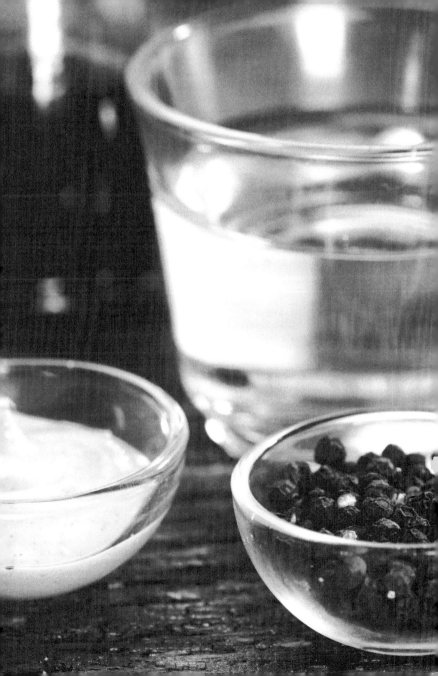

GARLIC OIL

NUT-FREE, VEGETARIAN, VEGAN, PALEO-FRIENDLY, DAIRY-FREE, SOY-FREE

Makes 1 cup. Prep time: 5 minutes, plus 10 minutes to rest.
Cook time: 10 minutes

Garlic oil is used in several recipes throughout this book. While garlic contains FODMAPs, if you use it to flavor oil and then strain away all of the solids, it won't aggravate your IBS—but it will allow you to enjoy some garlic flavor.

1 cup extra-virgin olive oil   6 garlic cloves, sliced

1. Place the olive oil in a small saucepan over medium-low heat. Add the garlic and bring it to a simmer. Reduce the heat to low and simmer, stirring frequently, for 5 minutes.

2. Allow the oil to cool for at least 10 minutes, or longer for a stronger flavored oil. Strain the oil through a fine-mesh sieve and discard the solids.

3. Store the oil in a tightly sealed container in the refrigerator for up to 1 week.

Per Serving (1 tablespoon) Calories 120; Protein 0g; Sugar 0g; Fat 14g

Books, Apps, and Websites

The following resources will help you stay abreast of the latest low-FODMAP research.

Books

IBS-Free at Last! Change Your Carbs, Change Your Life with the FODMAP Elimination Diet
by Patsy Catsos

This comprehensive self-help book is designed to provide instruction on how to implement a low-FODMAP diet to relieve the symptoms of IBS. The book explains FODMAPs in an easy-to-understand manner and provides a diet that looks relatively simple to follow.

Features:
- Lists of foods to enjoy and foods to avoid
- A step-by-step plan
- An explanation of the science behind the low-FODMAP diet
- Meal plans

I Have IBS...Now What?!!!
by Ashkan Farhadi

This is a small book that is a must read for anyone who is suffering from IBS. The author is a hands-on gastroenterologist at Rush University Medical Center in Chicago who treats people with IBS and other gastrointestinal diseases and conditions. Farhadi is also a researcher into IBS.

Features:
- An easy-to-understand explanation of IBS
- Triggers and possible causes of IBS
- Research into IBS
- Symptoms of IBS
- Treatment options
- How to get a diagnosis
- Tips to find relief of symptoms

The Low-FODMAP Diet Cookbook by Sue Shepherd

This is a companion book for *The Complete Low-FODMAP Diet*. Dr. Shepherd is the originator of the low-FODMAP diet. There is some explanation about the low-FODMAP diet in scientific terms, but the book is mostly a well-designed cookbook that provides choices for people who want to eat well without triggering IBS symptoms.

Features:

- A summary of the low-FODMAPs diet
- An explanation of other conditions or diseases that might be positively impacted by the diet
- An assortment of recipes for all levels of culinary skill, covering all courses, including dessert
- Vegan and vegetarian recipes and adaptions

The Complete Low-FODMAP Diet by Sue Shepherd and Peter Gibson

The authors of this book were key participants in the research that pinpointed that a low-FODMAPs diet could provide relief from the symptoms of IBS. This book outlines a plan that seems less like a deprivation diet and more like a solution to a common condition.

Features:

- An explanation of the science behind the low-FODMAP diet
- Lists of foods to enjoy and foods to avoid
- Meal plans
- Recipes covering all courses and meals
- Practical tips pertinent to real life
- Research statistics behind the plan

Eating for IBS
by Heather Van Vorous

This is a cookbook written by someone who suffers from IBS and who shares the recipes that provided relief without being stingy on taste or variety. The author is a cook with her own TV show *Heather Cooks!* and a website designed to assist people dealing with IBS.

Features:

- Scientific statistics and research findings showing how the digestive system is affected by food
- An assortment of nutritious recipes, ranging from simple to complex
- A list of trigger foods and strategies to avoid them
- A general adherence to healthy eating guidelines that make the recipes in the book appropriate for anyone looking to live and eat well

App

Monash University's Low-FODMAP Diet App
http://www.lowfodmap.com /monash-university-fodmap -diet-app

The Monash University Low-FODMAP diet app is created from the work done at Monash University, where the early groundbreaking research was conducted on the effects of diet on IBS patients. This app was created in the wake of a high demand to pinpoint and understand FODMAPs in daily meals and be able to make educated choices about what to eat without experiencing IBS symptoms. The application places accurate information right at the user's fingertips whenever it is needed. This app is updated with the latest research and recommendations every twelve months.

Features:

- A copy of the Monash University low-FODMAP diet patient information booklet
- Articles about the low-FODMAP diet
- A food guide outlining foods to enjoy and foods to avoid in a searchable, color-coded format
- Appropriate serving sizes for each food
- Tips for following the diet
- Menu plans
- Recipes
- Shopping list templates
- Recipe recommendations in a seven-day challenge
- A symptom tracker template

Websites

IBS Diets FODMAP Dieting Guide
www.ibsdiets.org/fodmap-diet
/fodmap-food-list

Monash University's Low-FODMAP Diet for Irritable Bowel Syndrome
http://www.med.monash.edu/cecs
/gastro/fodmap

Kate Scarlata's IBS, FODMAP Diet, Celiac, and Diabetes Counseling Site
http://www.katescarlata.com

Shepherd Works Low-FODMAP Diet
http://shepherdworks.com.au
/disease-information
/low-fodmap-diet

–http://fodmapliving.com
/the-science/stanford
-university-low-fodmap-diet/

REFERENCES
Books and Other Sources

De Roest, R. H., B. R. Dobbs, B. A. Chapman, B. Batman, L. A. O'Brien, J. A. Leeper, C. R. Hebblewaite, and R. B. Gearry. "The Low-FODMAP Diet Improves Gastrointestinal Symptoms in Patients with Irritable Bowel Syndrome: A Prospective Study." *The International Journal of Clinical Practice* 67, no. 9 (May 2013): 895–903. doi:10.1111/ijcp.12128.

Environmental Working Group. "EWG's 2014 Shopper's Guide to Pesticides in Produce." Accessed May 14, 2014. http://www.ewg.org/release/ewgs-2014-shoppers-guide -pesticides-produce.

Hyman, Mark. "Three Hidden Ways Wheat Makes You Fat." *Huffington Post.* Last modified April 19, 2012. http://www.huffingtonpost.com/dr-mark-hyman/wheat -gluten_b_1274872.html.

International Foundation for Functional and Gastrointestinal Disorders. "Facts about IBS." Accessed May 6, 2014. http://www.aboutibs.org/site/what-is-ibs/facts.

Li, James T. C. "Diseases and Conditions: Food Allergy: What's the Difference Between a Food Intolerance and a Food Allergy?" Mayo Clinic. Accessed May 6, 2014.

http://www.mayoclinic.org/diseases-conditions/food-allergy
/expert-answers/food-allergy/faq-20058538.

Mayo Clinic. "Diseases and Conditions: Inflammatory Bowel
Disease." Accessed May 6, 2014. http://www.mayoclinic.org
/diseases-conditions/inflammatory-bowel-disease/basics
/definition/con-20034908.

National Foundation for Celiac Awareness. "Celiac Disease
Fast Facts." Accessed May 6, 2014. http://www.celiaccentral
.org/celiac-disease/facts-and-figures.

Stanford Hospitals & Clinics. "The Low-FODMAP Diet."
Accessed May 6, 2014. http://fodmapliving.com/wp-content
/uploads/2013/02/Stanford-University-Low-FODMAP
-Diet-Handout.pdf.

Sui, Yali, Gordana Djuras, and Gerhard M. Kostner. "Fructose
Malabsorption Influences Chronic and Recurrent Infectious
Diseases, Dyspepsia, and Heartburn." *The Open Gastroen-
terology Journal* 6 (2012): 1–7. Accessed May 6, 2014. http://
benthamscience.com/open/togasj/articles/V006
/1TOGASJ.pdf.

Thomas, J. Reggie, Rakesha Nanda, and Lin H. Shu. "A
FODMAP Diet Update: Craze or Credible?" *Practical Gastro-
enterology* (December 2012): 37–46. http://www.medicine.
virginia.edu/clinical/departments/medicine/divisions/diges-
tive-health/nutrition-support-team/nutrition-articles/Parrish
_Dec_12.pdf.

WebMD. "Irritable Bowel Syndrome (IBS) Health Center: Irritable Bowel Syndrome (IBS) Triggers and Prevention." Accessed May 6, 2014. http://www.webmd.com/ibs/guide /ibs-triggers-prevention-strategies.]

The Dirty Dozen
and the Clean Fifteen

The Dirty Dozen

APPLE

STRAWBERRY

GRAPE

CELERY

PEACH

SPINACH

SWEET BELL PEPPER

IMPORTED NECTARINE

CUCUMBER

CHERRY TOMATO

SNAP PEA

POTATO

The Clean Fifteen

ASPARAGUS

AVOCADO

CABBAGE

CANTALOUPE

CORN

EGGPLANT

GRAPEFRUIT

KIWI

MANGO

MUSHROOM

ONIONS

PAPAYA

PINEAPPLE

SWEET PEAS (FROZEN)

SWEET POTATO

CPSIA information can be obtained at www.ICGtesting.com
Printed in the USA
LVOW01s1155150315

430099LV00012BA/33/P